Yoga on HORSEBACK

A guide to mounted yoga exercises for riders

Nicole C. Cuomo, MA, OTR/L, RYT

Marty Whittle, ARIA Certified Instructor

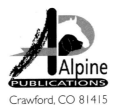

Alpine
PUBLICATIONS

Crawford, CO 81415

Yoga on Horseback: A guide to mounted yoga exercises for riders

Cataloging in Publication

Cuomo, Nicole C., 1965-
    Yoga on horseback : a guide to mounted yoga exercises for riders / Nicole C. Cuomo,
Martha Whittle.
        p. cm.
    ISBN 1-57779-080-4 (pbk.)
    1. Horsemanship. 2. Hatha yoga. I. Whittle, Martha, 1961-   II. Title
SF309.C86 2006
613.7'046—dc22

                                                                2006042886

The information contained in this book is complete and accurate to the best of our knowledge. All recommendations are made without guarantee on the part of the author or Alpine Publications, Inc. The author and publisher disclaim any liability with the use of this information. Neither the authors nor the publisher are liable for any damage caused or alleged to be caused directly or indirectly by the information contained in this book.

For the sake of simplicity, the terms "he" or "she" are sometimes used to identify an animal or person. These are used in the generic sense only. No discrimination of any kind is intended toward either sex.

This book is available at special quantity discounts for breeders and for club promotions, premiums, or educational use. Write for details.

Design: Laura Newport
Photos: Penny Barsch
Editing: Deb Helmers

1 2 3 4 5 6 7 8 9 0

Printed in the United States of America.

CONTENTS

ACKNOWLEDGMENTS

I would like to thank my husband Doug, friends and family members for their encouragement and support, and especially my son Neal, who knew when to take a long nap so that I could do some editing. I would also like to thank Lex, Stan and Johanna from the Yoga Institute and the Austin Yogashala for their guidance and teachings. Thanks to Marty for educating me on the importance of horsemanship and what it is to have a *good seat*. Peace.

—Nicole

I would like to thank my dearest Sal and my family and friends for their love and enthusiasm about the book. Many thanks to Nicole for introducing me to the wonders of yoga—it has enriched my life, riding and teaching immeasurably. My horses and teachers abound and I am eternally grateful for their patience, love and trust and their invaluable life lessons, past, present and future.

—Marty

We would both like to thank Penny Barsch for her time and the beautiful photographs. Great job, Penny, we really appreciate it!

Special thanks also go out to our equine models, Theodore (Teddy) and Miss Molly, for their patience, cooperation and understanding.

INTRODUCTION

HOW YOGA AIDS HORSEMANSHIP

This book is intended to open up your awareness of your own body as well as that of your horse. Through the practice of yoga, you develop balance, overall awareness, strength and flexibility. Once recognized, your vertical energy and your horse's horizontal energy can be combined in harmony.

Perhaps you share one of these typical trouble spots seen in riders:

- Fixing at the neck, shoulders and elbows
- An unbalanced, rigid seat, which can resist the horse's natural movement
- Sitting on the sacrum rather than on the seat bones
- Collapsing or rounding the chest forward
- Locking of the hips, knees and ankles

Through proper stretching and training, you can achieve:

- Elastic extension of the arms to permit movement through the reins and allow a receiving hand, which maintains contact with your horse's mouth while giving him freedom of the head, neck and back
- A relaxed seat, resulting in the ability to flow with your horse's movement
- A seat originating from the seat bones, which allows for movement of the pelvis and provides a balance point and base for the rest of your body
- An open chest, which keeps your hips and shoulders open and free-moving, making it easier to breathe
- Hips, knees and ankles that act as shock absorbers
- The ability to use your breath to promote awareness and focus

Did you ever hear something like: *The more you know, the more you realize how much you don't know?* Riding and yoga are lifelong learning practices—there is no point at which you can sit back and congratulate yourself on having learned all there is to know. Both riding and yoga often look easy to the lay person. Many of our students have complained, "It looks easy when you do it, but it's not," or "How can you make that look so easy?"

You cannot simply sit on a horse or stand on a yoga mat. In both practices, you must focus on body alignment, body awareness and the ability to stabilize one body part while moving another. Both riding and yoga require a focused mind; both are physically and mentally challenging. Both require correct breathing and movement. When riding, the more freely you move and breathe on top of your horse, the more freely your horse moves and breathes underneath you. Both practices also maintain a beautiful balance between strength and flexibility. It is possible to be very strong with little flexibility or very flexible with little strength, but when the correct balance is achieved, movement is strong, fluid and rhythmical.

Yoga and riding are forms of art in movement. They are both about balance, strength and flexibility, with a focused mind and an awareness of the here and now. Balance can be described as a combination of effort and the ability to surrender. Effort without surrender causes rigidity and can create a loss of sensitivity and awareness.

Yoga postures often focus on opening up the hips, chest and heart; these are all areas that are important when riding a horse.

We hope that the postures and exercises given here will improve your physical and emotional relationships with your horse. We also hope that you approach riding, yoga and your horse with dignity, compassion and an open heart and the postures with persistence and enthusiasm.

INJURY PREVENTION

Many injuries are due to a loss of focus. Losing focus leads to a separation of the mind, body and spirit. Fear, resistance, tension and fatigue all may bring about the loss of focus. We often hold our breath during times of physical and emotional stress, yet it is during these very times that that breathing and connecting is most important. With yoga and riding, we engage our muscles and breathe into the sensations that we feel. As distractions arise, it is important to bring awareness back to breathing. Breathing into the sensation promotes union of the body, mind and spirit, giving a sense of harmony, which in turn leads to muscle relaxation. Relaxation allows for muscle lengthening and allows the body to flow and balance.

Since every "body" is unique, it is important that you work within your own physical capability. Be kind to your body. And, as when beginning any exercise program, you should have your medical or health care professional's approval.

Chapter 1

Yoga Foundations and Guidelines for Practice

Yoga has been practiced for thousands of years. *Yoga* is a Sanskrit word meaning to yoke up or unite. Numerous books have been written on the different kinds of yoga; there are ancient texts, western interpretations and contemporary practices. The yoga introduction given here is a simplistic way of explaining a very deep and spiritual practice. In no way do we intend to educate you on all aspects of yoga, but, rather, we are merely giving a general explanation. At the back of this book, we provide a glossary of basic yoga terms. The first time these terms are used in this text, they appear in bold type. If you would like to begin a serious practice of yoga, you should find a certified yoga teacher in your area. A list of suggested readings is included in the bibliography at the end of this book.

TYPES OF YOGA

There are two basic categories of yoga. **Hatha** yoga (*hatha* meaning determined effort) is a type of yoga that works from the outside in. This yoga can be quite physical, including movement, breathing and stretching. It is also the yoga of energy intake and output, and focuses on your becoming aware of what type of energy you take in and send out into the world. Hatha yoga uses **mantras**, which are sound vibrations that can be either audible or silent; these vibrations give the mind an anchor and help decrease distraction and promote awareness. This type of yoga may also include the practice of love and devotion, which can include prayer or song.

Raja yoga is known as mind yoga, the type of yoga that works from the inside out. **Patanjali's Yoga Sutras** (threads of knowledge), approximately two hundred steps to becoming a free being, is a type of mind yoga that leads to the path of **samadhi** (bliss or union with god). Raja yoga also includes **karma** yoga, where you become fully conscious of your actions rather than being focused on outcomes.

For the purposes of this book, we will be focusing mostly on hatha yoga, or the yoga of physical movement, stretching and breathing, although the raja yoga principle of working from the mind out is important and will be discussed briefly.

Yoga is the union of body, mind and spirit. The practice should be explored with an open heart and mind. Strive to become aware and refrain from judging. Use your mind for observations and possibilities, and allow yourself to move towards new pathways to balance, serenity and freedom of movement.

YOGA BASICS

- Practice on an empty stomach, or have a piece of fruit or glass of juice; it is best to wait approximately two hours after a large meal before practicing yoga.
- Practice barefoot in comfortable (stretchable) clothing.
- If you have a history of pain or other health concerns, contact a certified yoga teacher for assistance in proper alignment and variations of the postures.
- Be gentle with yourself. Some postures may be difficult depending on your body's current ability to stretch and lengthen. Being gentle and accepting can go a long way in helping your progress.
- For the mounted postures, it is suggested that you wear safety attire, such as boots with a heel and an approved helmet (by ASTM/SEI, the American Standard for Testing Materials and Safety Equipment Institute). It is suggested that you have someone assist in holding your horse, or work with an ARIA, BHSA or NARHA certified instructor or educated horseperson.
- Breathe, breathe, breathe.

Chapter 2

Yoga, Riding and Breathing

Prana is a vital energy; it can be explained as life's breath, or that which sustains life. Pranayama is the prolongation or extension and retention of breath, practiced in order to enable concentration and to regulate thoughts. Breath control should be performed gently, since overcontrolling or forcing the breath can lead to rigidity in breathing and the fixing or stabilizing of patterns in the body, as well as to an uneasiness of the mind.

In order to begin, one must first bring awareness to the breath. Following your breathing patterns is a way of becoming aware of your breath and also is the beginning of meditation.

BASICS OF BREATHING

- Breathing in and out (inhalation/exhalation) mainly arises from movement of the diaphragm. The diaphragm is a dome-shaped, musculomembranous partition, which moves down and out on inhalation and up and in on exhalation.
- Accessory muscles in your upper chest area and between your ribs assist in inhalation/exhalation.

- The breath expands in all directions and slightly moves the whole body.
- Poor posture (stooping forward, rounded shoulders, etc.) interferes with the effectiveness of breathing.

BRINGING AWARENESS TO YOUR BREATH

- Lie on your back with your hands on your diaphragm (at the edge of your rib cage), close your eyes, and let your breath come and go in a natural pattern. Feel your diaphragm rise and fall with each breath. Move your hands to your clavicles (collarbones) and feel the slight movement of your upper chest as you breathe in and out.
- Sit (either in a chair with your feet on the floor or on the floor on a meditation cushion or pillow with your legs crossed) with a straight back so that your waist is rising up and out of your hips. Let your abdomen and shoulders be soft (free from tension). Again, feel the movement of your diaphragm as you breathe in and out.

Combining Breath and Movement

A basic component to yoga and horseback riding is the ability to combine breath with movement. You will initially begin with small movements; then you will combine breath and movement in the postures (**asanas**). This will be the foundation of using breathing techniques when performing the mounted exercises. To start:

- Sit on a chair or a cushion and extend your back upward so that you are lifting up and out of your pelvis with a soft abdomen and shoulders.
- Inhale and raise your arms, palms up and open, so that your arms are out away from your body and your shoulder blades can slide down your back. As you inhale, lengthen your spine.
- Exhale, bring your hands to your legs, and slightly round your shoulders and look downwards.
- Repeat this breath 4-6 times.

The Complete Breath

- Sit either on a chair or a cushion on the floor, and exhale slowly through your nose.
- Begin the sequence by slowly inhaling through the nose, breathing into your upper chest/clavicle area and continuing to inhale as you expand your ribs and finally your abdomen.
- Exhale through your nose, initiating the movement from your abdomen.
- Repeat the sequence 6-10 times.
- If you feel dizzy, bring your breathing back to your normal pattern for a few breaths.

By breathing into the upper chest and expanding the air into the ribs and abdomen, you essentially cause a bellows effect, ensuring that air is being delivered into all areas of the lungs.

Nadi Sodhana (alternate nostril breath)

Nadis are energy channels which allow for the passage of prana. Sodhana means purifying. So **nadi sodhana** can be described as a purification of the energy or nerves; it creates a sense of calm and helps to focus the mind.

- Sit comfortably (chair or pillow).
- Rest your left hand on your lap or left thigh.
- Position your right hand so that your thumb, ring and pinky finger are extended and your index and middle fingers are curled into your palm.

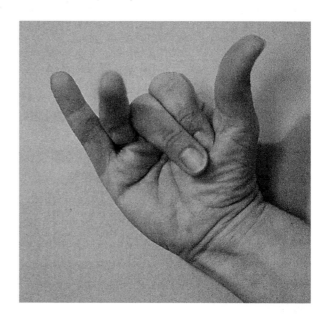

- Place your thumb to the outside of your right nostril, and then close your right nostril and breathe into your left nostril.
- Close your left nostril with your ring and pinky fingers, and release (open) your right nostril and exhale.
- Inhale through your right nostril; then open your left nostril and exhale.

You have just completed one round. Complete 4-6 rounds and slowly increase as you become more comfortable.

BREATHING AND RIDING

Holding your breath can cause tension throughout your own body and that of your horse. Your back muscles tighten and your base of support narrows. Holding your breath also causes you to become tired and winded easily. Breath-holding can also bring about uneven and off-balance transitions.

When you allow your diaphragm to expand and open during inhalation and then come up and in during exhalation, you are ensuring that you have enough breath for whatever the task at hand is. Steady, even breathing can be coordinated into the horse's gait to produce a fluidity of motion in the horse and the rider. As you use your breath, you create a gentler, more balanced posture, which allows the horse to move and breathe with greater ease. Breath-holding or sharp, narrow breathing can create tension in your shoulders, seat and legs. To compare, try gait transitions while holding your breath, and then try them while exhaling.

Listen to your horse's breathing as you coordinate your own breath into the gait. A paired rhythm of gait and breath encourages the natural pattern of the horse's breath as well. An audible breath or deep sigh can release tension and confusion in both you and your horse. This is an excellent tool to use when you have reached an awkward or resistant place in training.

Chapter 3

Riding and Meditation

The question of how mind and body mutually affect each other is an age-old one. The topic has experienced a broad range of publicity over the last few years, and examples of both positive and negative effects abound. For our purposes, we want to consider how your ability to focus and concentrate, and your emotions, affect your ride. Let's face it, we all have good and bad days. Some days we amaze ourselves; other days we may decide to just start knitting. A calm and focused mind can do a lot towards being successful in any arena of life. Meditation is a path towards acceptance of ourselves as we are, and it allows us to participate actively in our lives rather than reactively or as a reflection.

One of the simplest forms of meditation can be called "following the breath." In a seated position (either in a chair with both feet on the floor or on a cushion on the floor), begin by assuming a posture indicative of dignity and conviction. Lift your waist up out of your hips and your shoulders up out of your waist. Let your stomach, shoulders, neck and face be soft. Allow your breathing to be natural, not controlled in any way; let your eyes close, and pair the word "rising" with your inhalation and the word "falling" with your exhalation. If you become distracted by thoughts, sensations or sounds in the environment, bring yourself back to your breath using the words "rising" and "falling." Begin by sitting for just a few minutes, and slowly increase your meditation time to 10 minutes, 15 minutes and then 30 minutes. It is often difficult at first to sit and focus on your breath; it does, however, become easier.

A mantra is the repetition of a sound or phrase that helps to anchor the mind, such as "I am peaceful," "I am calm," or "I am fluid." A few minutes of meditation before you ride, whether for a hack, for a lesson or before a show, can help you focus and find peace and balance. If you are interested in finding out more about meditation, join a local meditation group or a yoga and meditation class.

Chapter 4

Un-Mounted Yoga Postures

The un-mounted exercises are designed to give you an understanding of how your body moves when you use breath and awareness as an anchor. The postures included in this section were chosen to give you a basic understanding of the mounted postures, as well as to introduce some basic yoga postures designed to open up your shoulders and hips, increase your spinal flexibility, and improve your balance. These postures are influenced by the **ashtanga** and **viniyoga** branches of yoga. First you will move in and out of the postures, which fosters flexibility and enhances the learning process. (After all, humans are not static beings.) Once you have moved in and out of a particular posture, you may stay longer in it, using your breath as a focus and support. Staying in a posture fosters strength as well as patience. Again, it is recommended that you have your medical or health care professional's approval before beginning any exercise program.

It is important to keep in mind that we all work with different levels of strength and flexibility. You must be honest with yourself and cognizant of working within your own limitations. One of the yoga sutras, **sthirasukhamasanam** (sutra II.46), translates as: *Yoga postures should be comfortable and stable; a posture that causes pain or restlessness is* *not a yogic posture.* Work within your own spectrum of strength and flexibility, and allow yourself to perform the posture as best as you can. Although strength and flexibility vary widely from person to person and often decline with age, the benefits yoga offers do not depend on perfect execution of the postures. Indeed, the "perfect" position is often unattainable for the novice and experienced practitioner alike. So don't let yourself be discouraged by a less-than-perfect performance; instead, focus on what you *can* accomplish.

ALIGNMENT

You will find that many of the postures benefit all areas of your body. The following will look at proper alignment and its importance, working from the top of your head to your feet.

Head, Neck and Eyes

The head is balanced by your neck; any displacement of the head and neck will affect your spinal alignment. Your goal is to carry your head erect with soft and accepting eyes and neck muscles.

This means not fixing your eyes or tightening the muscles of your neck and face.

Shoulders and Arms

Tightness around the shoulder muscles is common; most of us hold tension and unevenness in our shoulders. The shoulder area includes the upper back, scapula (shoulder blade), clavicle (collarbone) and humerus (upper arm bone). Your goal is to open your chest and inflate the front of your body, allowing you to relax and giving freedom to the lower back and pelvis. It is through relaxed shoulders that your arms are able to move when holding the reins without locking at the elbow.

Abdomen

This is the area of physiological centering, balance and strength. Your goal is to be able to keep an erect posture while allowing movement through the hips and lower back. A toned abdomen allows you to keep your pelvis neutral with a slight posterior tilt without locking the hips and lower back.

Lower Back and Pelvis

The lower back (lumbar spine) articulates with the sacrum (five fused spinal bones). Your goal is to be able to sit in the saddle with loose hips and pelvis so that you move with the horse. Tipping your pelvis too far forward (anterior pelvic tilt) or too far back (posterior pelvic tilt) locks the hips and legs, which can cause discomfort for both you and your horse.

Legs

The femur (thigh bone) must be able to rotate inward to allow you to sit comfortably in a saddle. Your goal is a balance between leg strength and flexibility, in order to feel secure in the saddle. A secure lower leg against the horse provides communication to the horse and stability for the rest of your body.

BEGINNING THE POSTURES

In order to enhance learning, it is imperative that you practice and repeat the postures. If you are not working with a qualified yoga teacher, ask a friend or use a mirror to check your alignment. Begin slowly until you are comfortable with the movements, and work within your own range of movement and flexibility.

Once you learn the postures, you can focus on specific areas you feel you need to work on or you can mix up the sequence. At the end of the chapter are suggested practice sequences both for beginners and for those with experience. It is important to remember that you should always begin with a warm-up and end with a period of relaxation or meditation.

Please note: If you feel dizzy or short of breath, it generally means you have pushed yourself too far too fast, and you should rest, either sitting or in Relaxation. If a posture feels uncomfortable, it is usually your body telling you that something is not right. If you do feel you need to come out of a posture to rest, do so

Always begin your yoga session with a warm-up and end it with a period of relaxation or meditation.

slowly and gently and make sure that you are breathing correctly. Keep in mind that you can be your own best friend as well as your own worst enemy—listen to your body, so that you will know when to persist and when to rest. If you ignore the signals that something is wrong or uncomfortable, you may wind up injured.

We recommend that you review all the postures prior to attempting them and seek advice if you are unclear about any of them.

WARM-UPS

Warm ups are designed to prepare the body for more challenging postures. It is important to increase the blood flow to the large muscle groups prior to putting demands on them. Warming up the muscles helps protect you from muscle injury and soreness.

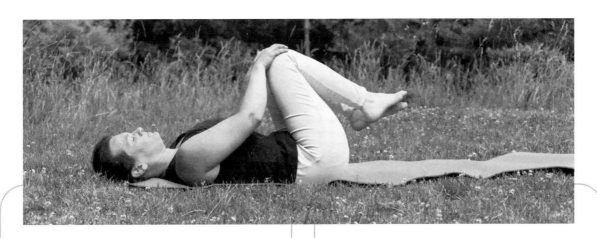

LOWER ABDOMEN 1

Allows the joints to realign themselves, lets heart and lungs rest; a good counterpose for many postures. Do not perform if you have sciatic nerve problems, unless you are working with a certified yoga teacher.

Begin by lying on your back with knees up and feet on the floor.

Exhale and lift your legs up, knees toward the chest. Place your hands on your knees.

Inhale and let your knees move away from your body.

Exhale and let your knees come closer.

Use your abdominal muscles, and let your hands simply rest on your knees, following the movement.

Repeat 6-10 times.

LOWER ABDOMEN 2

Allows the joints to realign themselves, lets heart and lungs rest; a good counterpose for many postures. Do not perform if you have sciatic nerve problems.

Begin by lying on your back with knees up and feet on the floor.

Exhale and lift your legs up, knees toward the chest. Place your hands on your knees.

Gently circle your knees clockwise.

Stop in the center.

Gently circle your knees counterclockwise.

Stop in the center.

Do 4-6 circles in each direction.

ROCK AND ROLL

Loosens the muscles in the shoulders, back and pelvis; also works the abdomen muscles.

Begin by sitting on the ground.

Cross your legs and hold onto the opposite shins or ankles with your hands.

Roll back and forth from the pelvis to the upper back, tucking the head into the chest slightly. Repeat 3-5 times.

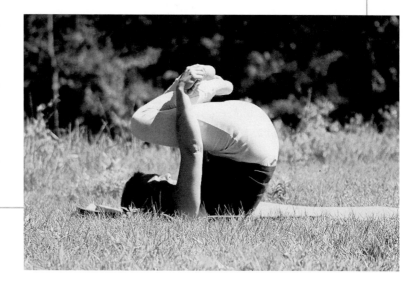

BRIDGE

Assists in learning proper breathing; the variations stretch the shoulders; a common counterpose.

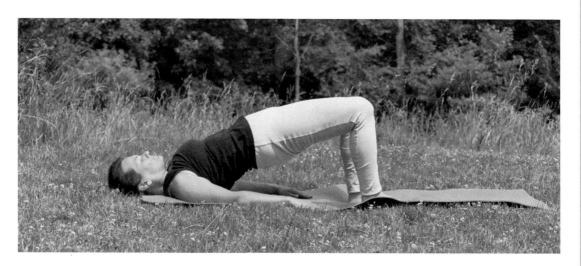

Lie on your back with knees bent, feet on floor under knees, heels together, and arms along your sides.

Exhale and slightly tip the pubic bone towards the navel.

Inhale and lift the pelvis, rolling up one vertebra at a time.

Exhale and lower down, one vertebra at a time.

Repeat 2-4 times. Then stay in raised pose for several breaths.

BRIDGE VARIATION 1

Inhale and lift the pelvis, one vertebra at a time, while raising the right arm over head to the floor.

Exhale and lower the pelvis, one vertebra at a time, while lowering the arm.

Inhale and lift the pelvis and the left arm over head.

Exhale and lower the pelvis and the arm.

Repeat 2-4 times each side.

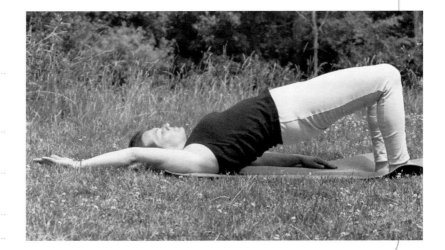

BRIDGE VARIATION 2

Inhale and lift the pelvis, raising both arms over head.

Exhale and lower the pelvis and the arms.

Repeat 2-4 times.

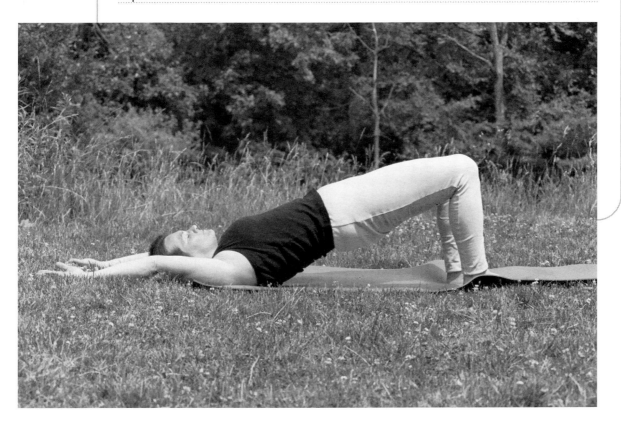

RUDDY GOOSE TO CHILD

A great warm-up asana used to strengthen and lengthen the back of the body; can also be used between other asanas as a counterpose.

Begin on your hands and knees (Ruddy Goose), with a slight tension in your hands as if you were sliding them backwards towards your feet; this will stabilize the shoulders and bring the scapula (shoulder blades) down your back.

Exhale and bring your hips towards your feet as you round your lower back, middle back and upper back until you are completely lowered.

Inhale and extend the upper back, middle back and lower back, leading with your shoulders and chest, while rising to your hands and knees.

Move in and out several times (6-10 times).

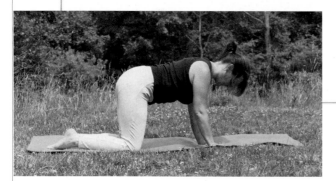 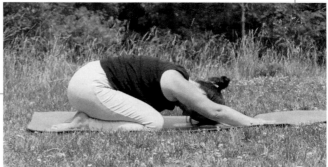

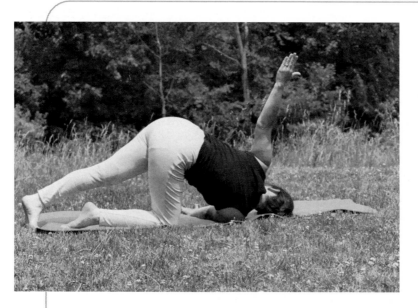

THREAD THE NEEDLE

Used to open up the shoulders and to provide a stretch to the sides of the body.

Begin on your hands and knees.

Inhale and raise your right arm up and out to the side.

Exhale and slowly lower your arm, threading it under your left arm.

Resting your right shoulder on the floor, inhale and raise your left arm up and turn to look up at your left hand.

If you feel balanced, extend your left leg out behind you, toes on the floor.

Stay for several breaths.

Inhale to come up.

Repeat to the other side.

Breathing Exercises

Complete breath and alternate nostril breathing, as described in Chapter 2.

STANDING AND KNEELING POSTURES

Note: *All standing poses begin and end in Mountain.*

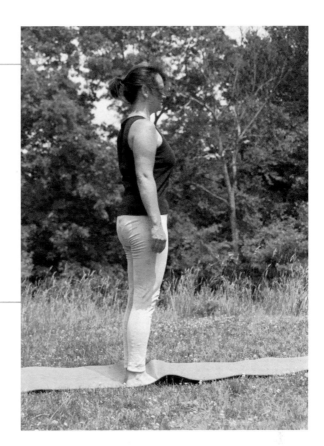

MOUNTAIN

Improves postural alignment, stability, balance and centering.

Stand with feet slightly apart and parallel, weight equally balanced on both feet.

Legs are straight; knees unlocked and slightly bent; chin slightly tucked, eyes open.

Abdomen is slightly drawn in to lessen lumbar curve (slight pelvic tuck).

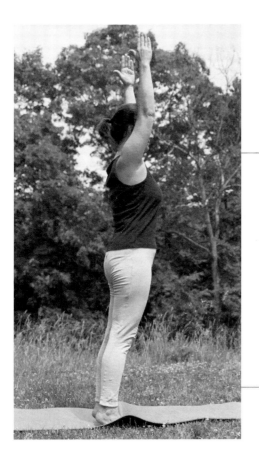

STRAIGHT TREE

Develops calmness, balance and strength.

Begin in Mountain.

Inhale and raise arms up over head while raising your heels so you are balancing on the balls of your feet. Only rise as high as you can without losing your balance.

Exhale and lower your arms and heels, returning to Mountain.

Repeat 2-6 times.

FORWARD FOLD

Stretches and strengthens spine, a relaxing posture that warms the body. Avoid staying in the posture if you have migraines, high blood pressure, sinus or ear or neck pain.

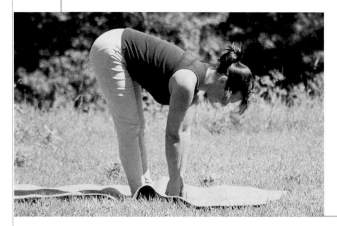

Begin in Mountain.

Inhale and raise arms up and over head.

Exhale, bend at hips, and with knees slightly bent, lower your body, relaxing the head and neck and letting the arms hang.

Place hands on thighs and inhale, tuck the chin and lift the upper back, middle back, then lower back (using the strength of your legs to push you up).

Repeat 2-6 times, and then stay for 2-4 breaths.

STANDING YOGA MUDRA — A **mudra** (literally, seal) is a symbolic gesture made with the hand or fingers.

Opens up the shoulders, stretches and strengthens the back. Avoid staying in the posture if you have migraines, high blood pressure, sinus or ear or neck pain.

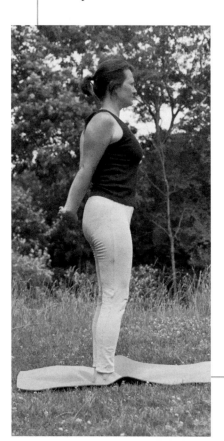

Begin in Mountain.

Inhale and raise your arms up and forward to chest level.

Exhale and bring your hands together behind your back, clasping them together (if you cannot clasp your hands together, hold on to a cloth or strap for the same effect).

Inhale and extend up, opening the front of your body.

Exhale and bend at the hips into a forward bend, knees slightly bent, and bring your clasped hands up behind your back.

Stay for several breaths.

Inhale as you rise up.

Exhale and release your hands.

Repeat 2-6 times.

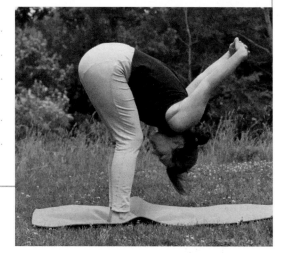

INTENSE STRETCH WITH FEET SPREAD

Increases circulation to the pelvic area, opens up the hip joints, develops breathing into the back of the body. Avoid staying in the posture if you have migraines, high blood pressure, sinus or ear or neck pain.

Begin in Mountain.

Step left foot out to the side, toes facing forward, feet parallel.

Inhale and extend the spine.

Exhale and bring hands to hips.

Inhale, and then exhale while bending forward at the hips, letting the knees bend slightly, place hands on floor.

Inhale and slide hands up legs as you straighten your upper back, middle back, then lower back, using the strength in your legs.

Move in and out of the posture 4-6 times, and then stay for 4 breaths.

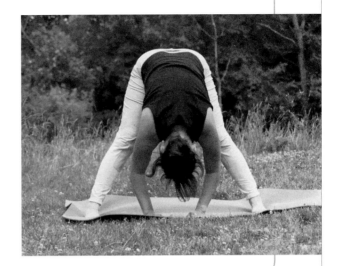

CHAIR

Develops thighs and knees, brings awareness to keeping weight in the heels. Do not do pose if it creates lasting pain in the knee.

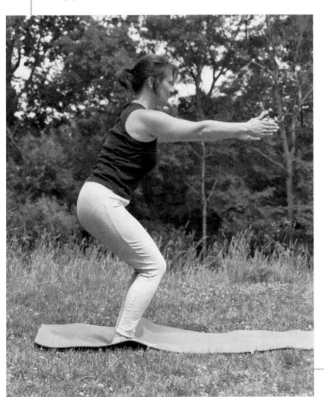

Begin in Mountain.

Inhale and raise arms over head.

Exhale, squat halfway down, keeping knees together and back straight, arms out in front at shoulder level. (You will be angled slightly forward.)

Keep shoulder blades down and back, and back straight.

Inhale and return to standing, using the strength of your legs, and raise arms over head.

Repeat 5-10 times, increasing the repetitions as you feel able, eventually working up to 5 sets of 5.

As you feel stronger, begin to stay in the position, starting with 4 breaths and working up to 8 breaths.

AWKWARD CHAIR — This is an advanced pose; begin once you can perform Chair with greater ease.

Develops thighs and knees, brings awareness to keeping weight in the heels; an excellent way to strengthen legs for the half-seat position and to feel the balance for a centered jumping position. Do not do pose if it creates lasting pain in the knee.

Exhale and squat halfway down, with weight in your heels.

Inhale and bring your hands together, palms facing each other in prayer fashion.

Exhale and twist to the left, placing the outside of the right shoulder to the outside of the left leg, keeping the knees even and weight in your heels.

Stay for several breaths, and then inhale and return to center.

Exhale.

Inhale and stand.

Repeat to the other side. For more advanced students, hold posture for 5-7 breaths.

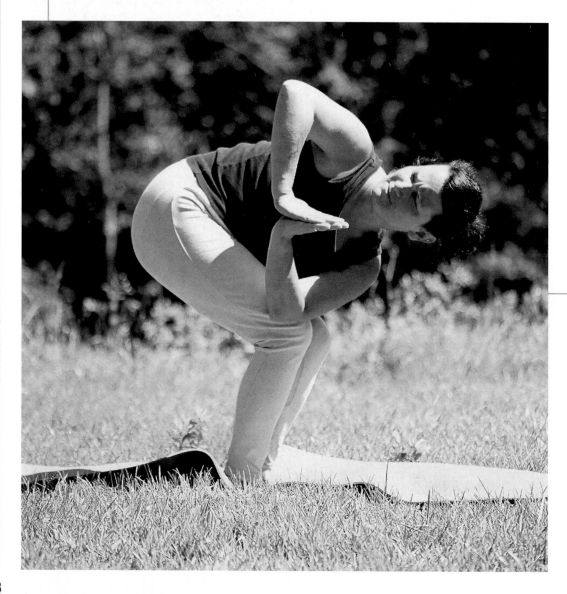

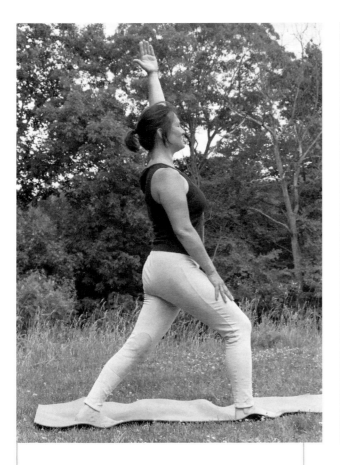

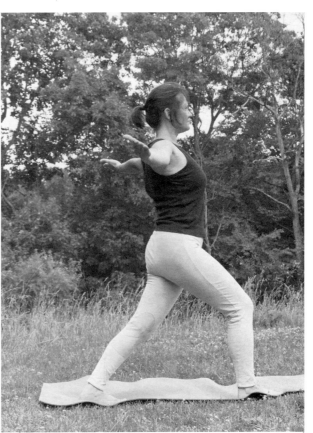

WARRIOR I

An upper-back bend that develops strength, breathing capacity and balance; helps to develop determination while strengthening the legs. Avoid staying in the posture if you have knee or ankle problems.

Begin in Mountain.

Step forward with your right foot, keeping feet apart, hips square.

Place your right hand on your right thigh.

Inhale and move forward and bend your right knee as you sweep your left arm out to the side and up over head.

Exhale and return to straight leg posture, bringing your arm down by your side.

Repeat 4-6 times, moving in and out of the posture, and then stay in the pose using deep breaths (4-6 breaths).

Repeat to the other side.

Then hold on each side for 2-6 breaths.

WARRIOR I VARIATION

An upper-back bend that develops strength, breathing capacity and balance; helps to develop determination while strengthening the legs. Avoid staying in the posture if you have knee or ankle problems.

Begin in Mountain.

Step forward with your right foot, keeping feet apart, hips square.

Inhale and raise your arms up and out to the sides, palms up.

Exhale and move forward and bend the right knee.

Inhale and return to straight leg posture.

Exhale and bring your arms down by your side.

Stay for 2-6 breaths.

Repeat to the other side.

WARRIOR 2

Opens up the groin area while strengthening the legs and back. Avoid if you have lower back problems.

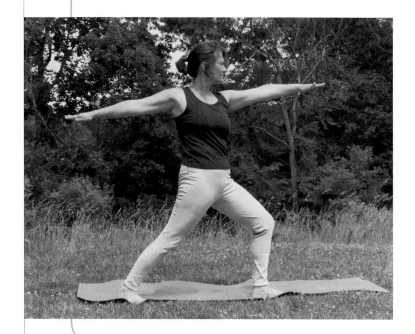

Begin in Mountain.

Step forward with your left foot. As you step, bring your right foot to a 45-degree angle, toes turning slightly out, but maintaining a slight inward rotation of your right leg.

Inhale and raise your arms, left arm forward and right arm behind you.

Exhale and bend the left knee, dropping your weight down and opening up the groin area.

Stay for 2-6 breaths.

Inhale and return to straight leg posture.

Exhale and bring legs together.

Repeat on the other side.

DOWNWARD DOG

Strengthens the arms and opens the rib cage, while stretching the back of the legs and lumbar spine. Avoid staying in posture if you have hypertension, migraines or neck, wrist or shoulder pain. Avoid posture if you have a heart condition, unless under supervision of a certified yoga teacher.

Begin on hands and knees (Ruddy Goose).

Curl the toes under.

Exhale and lead with the tailbone as you lift your body up and back. Keep your back straight and knees slightly bent (you can straighten your knees only if it has no consequence to a straight back).

Inhale and return to hands and knees.

Repeat, coming in and out of the posture 4-6 times, and then stay for 4-6 breaths.

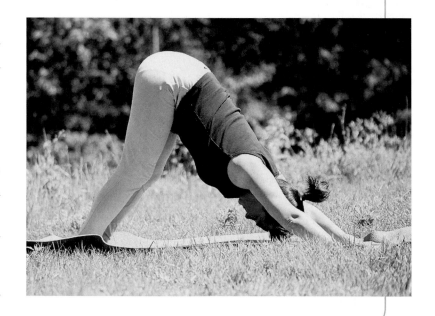

DOWNWARD DOG TO LUNGE

Strengthens the arms and opens the rib cage, while stretching the back of the legs and lumbar spine. Avoid staying in posture if you have hypertension, migraines or neck, wrist or shoulder pain.

From Downward Dog, inhale and step the left foot in between the hands into a lunge, keeping the shoulders open and back, and breathing into the belly.

Exhale and step back to Downward Dog.

Repeat to the other side.

Repeat 2-4 times each side, and then stay 2-4 breaths.

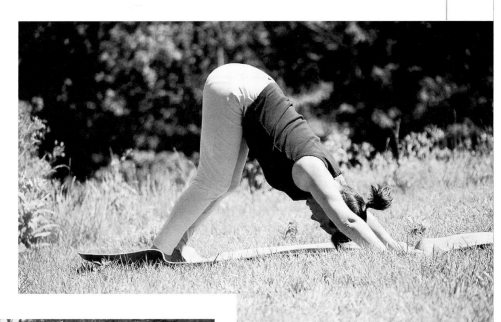

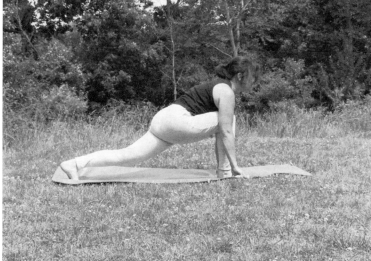

DOWNWARD DOG TO PIGEON

Opens hips and pelvis, strengthens arms and upper back. Avoid if you have sciatic nerve or knee pain or heart problems, unless under supervision of a certified yoga teacher.

Begin on hands and knees (Ruddy Goose).

Curl the toes under.

Exhale and lead with the tailbone as you lift your body up and back. Keep your back straight and knees slightly bent (you can straighten your knees only if it has no consequence to a straight back).

Inhale and lift your left leg straight back up off the floor.

Exhale and slide your left leg down and forward, dropping your knee and ankle (ankle under the right hip).

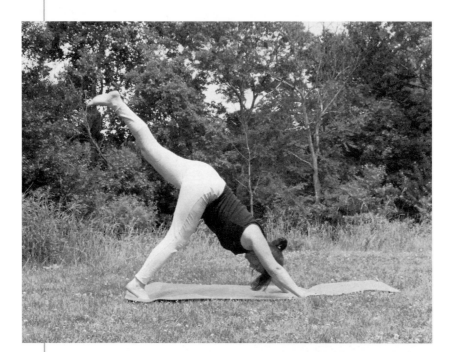

Exhale and lower down.

Inhale and extend your upper back, opening the chest. (Keep your hips as even as possible—don't let hips fall to one side.)

Stay for 2-6 breaths.

Exhale and bring your leg back under you to hands and knees; then slowly lower your lower back, middle back and upper back to Child.

Inhale to Ruddy Goose and repeat to the other side.

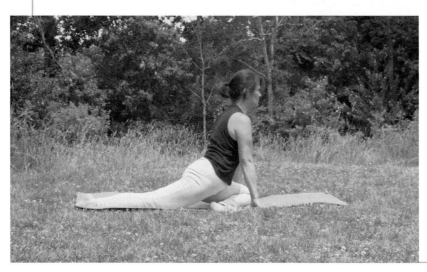

HALF CAMEL

Opens up the front of the body. Avoid if you have low back pain or a weak lower back.

Begin with tall kneeling, toes curled under.

Inhale and lift your left arm up over head.

Exhale, twist back and reach right hand to right ankle.

Inhale and return back to center.

Exhale and lower arm.

Repeat to right side.

Alternate 4-6 times on each side.

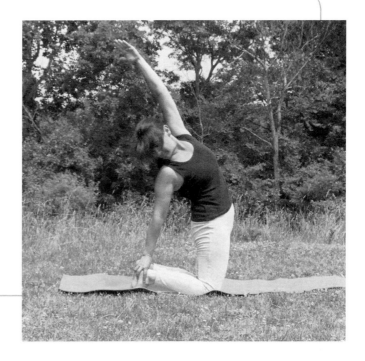

PRONE (FACE DOWN) POSTURES

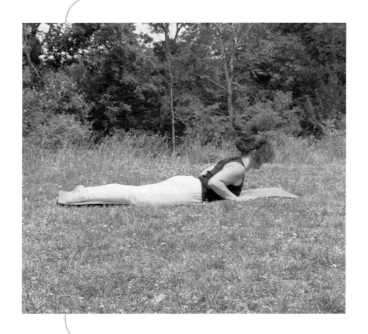

COBRA VARIATION

Strengthens and elongates the back of the body.

Begin on your stomach with your forehead touching the floor, your hands near your shoulders and your feet together.

Inhale and extend your upper back and chest, lifting them slightly off the ground.

Exhale and lower to the ground.

Move your feet apart slightly (about 1 inch) and repeat.

Continue for 5 more repetitions, moving your feet outwards a little farther each time; then reverse directions and continue until your legs are together.

SEATED POSTURES

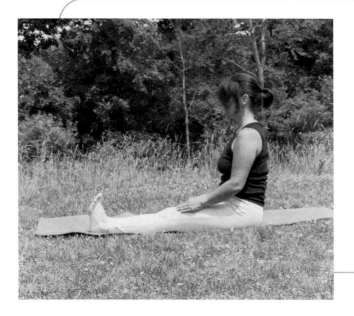

STICK

Strengthens the torso, stimulates deep breathing.

Sit with legs and back straight, chin slightly down and arms resting comfortably by your sides. (Sit on a cushion, pillow or rolled up blanket if you have low-back problems—this will keep your natural low back curve.)

Begin by staying for 2-4 breaths, and then work your way up to 6-8 breaths. If you have tight hamstring muscles, bend your knees slightly to keep your back straight.

HEAD TO KNEE

Strengthens the back, opens up the hip joint.

Begin in Stick.

Bend your right leg and place the sole of the foot in line with the opposite thigh, keeping your left leg extended straight in front of you.

Inhale and raise your arms over head.

Exhale and bend forward at the hips, bringing your arms down, hands toward your ankle. Keep seat bones parallel and back and pelvis straight.

Inhale and come up with your arms over head.

Move in and out 4-6 times, and then stay for 4-6 breaths.

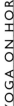

TABLE

Strengthens the shoulder girdle, hip, thighs and buttocks.

Begin in a seated position with legs bent at the hips and knees, feet in front, palms behind you with fingers pointing towards the toes.

Inhale and lift your body up, bringing the head in line with the spine.

Hold your head straight with a slight chin tuck (this is easier on your neck).

Exhale and lower body back to sitting.

Repeat, moving in and out 4-6 times, and then stay for 4-6 breaths.

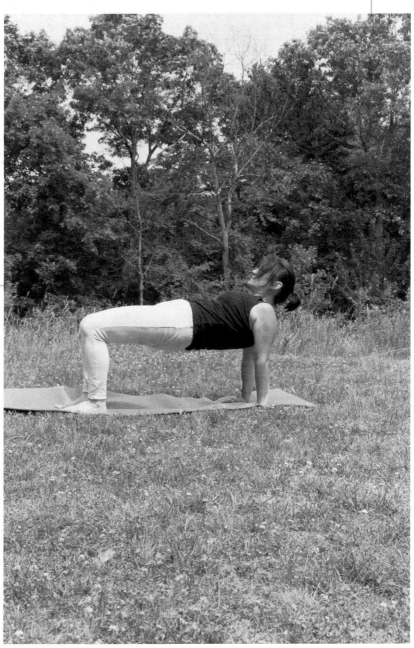

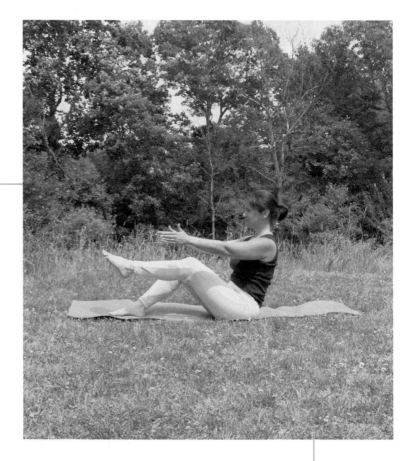

BOAT

Strengthens abdominal wall, hip flexors and lumbar spine.

Begin seated with knees bent and feet on floor in front of you.

Inhale and raise your arms out in front of your body at shoulder level.

Exhale and raise the left leg up with knee bent and lower leg parallel to floor.

Inhale and lower leg.

Exhale and raise right leg up.

Inhale and lower leg.

Repeat 2-4 times.

If and when you are ready, exhale and bring both legs up with knees bent and lower legs parallel to the floor, with your chest open and lifted.

Maintain your weight in your seat bones—don't rock back onto the sacrum.

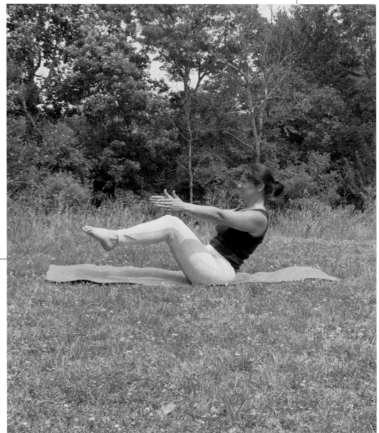

SEATED TWIST

Activates the abdominal area (solar plexus, digestive system) and stretches the muscles surrounding the spine.

Begin in Stick.

Fold the right leg under and place your left leg over your right leg with the left foot on the floor.

Inhale and extend the spine upwards (make yourself tall).

Exhale and twist to the left, wrapping your right arm over your left leg, turning your head and eyes to the left.

Inhale and return to center.

Repeat 2-4 times, and then stay for 4-6 breaths.

Repeat to the other side.

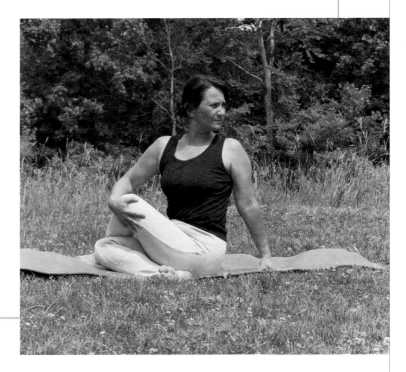

TAILOR

Stretches the inner thigh and groin. Avoid bending too far forward, as this could displace the sacral ligament.

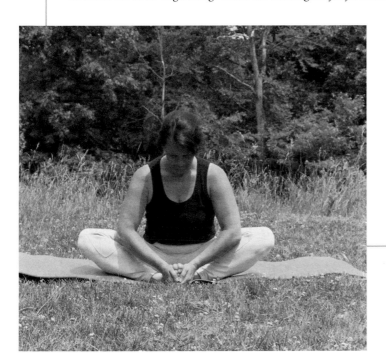

Begin seated with the soles of feet together in front of the groin.

Inhale and extend your spine upwards.

Exhale and bend slightly at the hips, keeping the back straight.

Breathe in and out deeply for several breaths.

Inhale and return to center.

INVERSIONS

Note: *The partial shoulder stand is as beneficial as a full shoulder stand, while being safer on the neck and back.*

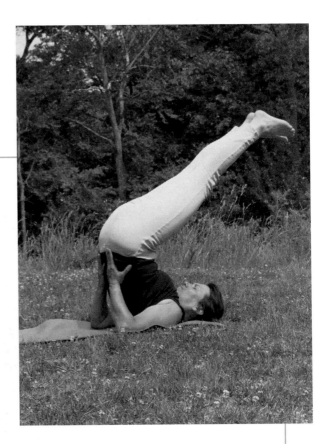

PARTIAL SHOULDER STAND

Strengthens abdomen and back. Contraindications are neck injuries, detached retina, glaucoma, migraines, pregnancy, high blood pressure and hiatal hernia.

Lie on your back, with your knees bent and feet on floor.

Lift your legs over your head, allowing the torso to come off the floor, and place your palms flat on the lower back.

Inhale and lift your legs slightly and breathe, keeping your toes relaxed.

Stay for 2-8 breaths, slowly working your way up to 16-20 breaths.

To come out, roll slowly down, bending the knees and hips until your back is on the floor.

COMPLETING THE PRACTICE

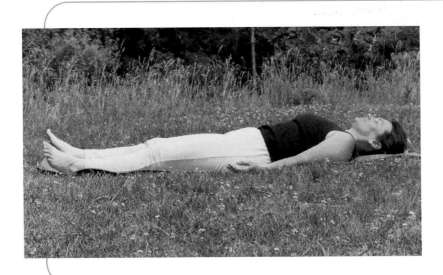

RELAXATION

Lie on your back with legs apart, feet relaxed, eyes closed, and head in a comfortable position.

Maintain proper spinal alignment while keeping muscles relaxed.

Give yourself time to sufficient time to relax. This can vary from 5-20 minutes, depending on your needs.

Relaxation Variations

If you have low-back problems, place a bolster towel or block under your knees. Soft music or mantras can help relax you while you are in this posture.

It is often easier to meditate after Relaxation, since you are then in a relaxed state with a clearer mind and are less likely to become internally distracted.

DAILY PRACTICE SUGGESTIONS

When beginning a home practice, it is essential to begin with warm-ups and to perform the postures within your own scope of strength and flexibility. You have to be patient and kind to yourself. Flexibility and strength will improve over time. Injuries occur when you are impatient or too forceful.

Find a space in your house or barn that is peaceful and uncluttered. If you can, leave your yoga mat there, along with any accessories that you use, such as straps, blankets or cushions and any meditation supplies. Try to find a time when you will be able to complete the practice uninterrupted, such as early in the morning or before bedtime. It depends on your own situation and responsibilities; you have to find a time that works for you.

PRACTICING ON A DAILY BASIS

With a busy schedule, it is often difficult to commit to a daily practice; however, if you can practice briefly every day, you will feel more balanced. Begin practice with a controlled breathing technique as described in Chapter 2. Begin the poses with one or two warm-up postures, and attempt to complete as many postures as you can, focusing on the areas where you need opening (such as hips or shoulders). Complete all practice sessions with at least five minutes of Relaxation.

If you find that you have a specific area of tightness, such as the shoulders, focus on the poses that open that area. You should include poses in standing, sitting and prone for an overall workout. Once you have experience with the following practice sequences, you will feel more confident in designing your own.

BEGINNER PRACTICES

The beginner practices are slightly gentler than those for the person experienced in yoga. It is a good idea to start with beginner sequences when you are new to yoga or new to a particular yoga style.

PRACTICE I

Lower Abdomen 1 and 2—4 x.

Bridge and Bridge variations—4 x each.

Ruddy Goose to Child—4 x

Mountain—2-4 breaths

Straight Tree—4 x

Forward Fold—2 x

Intense Stretch with Feet Spread—2 x

Chair—2-4 x

Warrior 1—2 x, then stay 2-4 breaths

Downward Dog—2 x, then stay 2-4 breaths

Cobra Variation—2-4 x

Seated Twist—2 x each side

Tailor—4-6 breaths

Relaxation—5-10 minutes

PRACTICE II

Ruddy Goose to Child—2-4 x

Bridge—2-4 x

Mountain—4 breaths

Straight Tree—2-4 x

Intense Stretch with Feet Spread—2 x

Chair—2-6 x

Warrior 2—2-4 breaths

Downward Dog—2-4 x, then stay 2-4 breaths

Downward Dog to Lunge—2 x each side

Stick (with pillow or knees bent)—2-4 breaths

Head to Knee—2 x each side

Table—2-4 x

Boat (1 leg at a time)—2 x each side

Tailor—2 x

Relaxation—5-10 minutes

EXPERIENCED PRACTICES

Once you are comfortable performing the beginner series, you can begin to practice more challenging poses.

PRACTICE I

Lower Abdomen 1 and 2—4-6 x.

Rock and Roll—2-4 x

Bridge and Bridge Variations—4-6 x each

Ruddy Goose to Child—4-6 x

Mountain—4-6 breaths

Straight Tree—4 x

Forward Fold—4-6 x, then stay 4-6 breaths

Standing Yoga Mudra—stay 2-4 breaths

Intense Stretch with Feet Spread—4 x, then stay 4-6 breaths

Chair—2-3 sets of 5, then stay 4-6 breaths

Warrior 1—2 x, then stay 2-4 breaths

Warrior 2—4-6 breaths

Downward Dog—2 x, then stay 2-4 breaths

Downward Dog to Pigeon—2-6 breaths each side

Cobra Variation—2-4 x, then stay 4-6 breaths

Seated Twist—2 x each side, then stay on each side 4-6 breaths

Tailor—4-6 breaths

Relaxation—5-10 minutes

PRACTICE II

Bridge Pose—2-4 x

Ruddy Goose to Child—2-4 x

Thread the Needle—4-6 breaths

Mountain—4-6 breaths

Straight Tree—2-4 x

Intense Stretch with Feet Spread—4 x, then stay 4-6 breaths

Chair—2-6 x

Awkward Chair—4-6 breaths each side

Warrior 1 Variation—2-4 x each side, then stay 4-6 breaths

Warrior 2—4-6 breaths each side

Downward Dog—2-4 x, then stay 4-6 breaths

Downward Dog to Lunge—2 x each side, then stay 4-6 breaths on each side

Stick (with pillow or knees bent)—2-4 breaths

Head to Knee—2 x each side, then stay 4-6 breaths each side

Table—2-4 x, then stay 4-6 breaths each side

Boat (1 leg at a time)—2 x each side, then both legs 4-6 breaths

Camel—2-4 breaths each side

Tailor—2 x, then stay 4-6 breaths

Relaxation—5-10 minutes

continued on next page. . .

PRACTICE III

Lower Abdomen 1 and 2—4-6 x

Rock and Roll—2-4 x

Bridge Pose—2-4 x, then stay 4-6 breaths

Mountain—4-6 breaths

Straight Tree—4 x

Forward Fold—4-6 x, then stay 4-6 breaths

Standing Yoga Mudra—2-6 breaths

Ruddy Goose to Child—2-6 x

Downward Dog—2-4 x, then stay 4-8 breaths

Downward Dog to Lunge—2 x each side, then stay 4-8 breaths on each side

Downward Dog—2 x, then stay 2-4 breaths

Downward Dog to Pigeon—2-8 breaths each side

Ruddy Goose to Child—2-4 x

Partial Shoulder Stand—10-12 breaths

Relaxation—5-10 minutes

Chapter 5

Mounted Exercises on the Lunge Line

Learning to ride on the lunge line has many benefits. Lunging enables you to focus on developing your legs and seat without having to think about steering your horse. A good seat requires maintenance through awareness, strength and flexibility. Working on the lunge line with a professional who has horse experience can be a rewarding experience for more advanced riders as well as new riders.

LUNGING KNOW-HOW

Lunge work should be carried out by a qualified instructor such as one certified by ARIA (American Riding Instructors Association), NARHA (North American Riding for the Handicapped Association) or BHS (British Horse Society), or by an educated horseman. The horse or pony used should be comfortable and sensible on the lunge in order to avoid injury. Your horse must be kind, gentle, levelheaded, trained to voice commands and preferably not too bouncy in the trot. He must be able to tolerate you moving about and stretching, so that you can focus on the breathing and movements of the poses. By trusting your horse

you can truly open up and absorb the feelings the stretches have to offer.

Lunging should take place in a ring or enclosed area, using a strong cotton lunge line free of knots. Use either a lunging caveson, or put the lunge line through the bit on the near side, over the head stall and attach it to the bit on the far side. This will allow you to control your horse's head. Use a light, flexible lunge whip six feet long with a six-foot lash. This will allow you to center yourself in a triangular position, so that you can stay between the horse's hip and head while lunging. If you do not feel comfortable lunging your horse safely, contact an instructor in your area for guidance.

Make sure you work on the lunge in both directions, as this allows you to balance and stretch both sides of your own and your horse's body—riders and horses all have one side that is stiffer. Before each session you can check in with yourself to determine which side of your body feels stiffer. Sit squarely in the saddle and relax into the bowl of your seat, letting each leg hang freely. Inhale and raise both arms up and out and twist to each side slowly, keeping the seat bones even in the saddle. Compare each side and determine which feels stiffer or less mobile. Begin the exercises by lunging to the side that feels stiffer.

It is also important to work with your horse at both the walk and the trot so that you can develop the body awareness and balance skills that you will need when riding on your own. Maintaining your posture, seat and lower leg will give you stability and allow your horse to move freely under you.

Remember the basic body concepts you worked on in the un-mounted postures:

- 🐾 Awareness of breath
- 🐾 Soft carriage of the head, neck and eyes
- 🐾 Open chest and front of body
- 🐾 Erect posture, using the abdominal muscles
- 🐾 Free movement through the hips and lower back
- 🐾 Balance between leg strength and flexibility

KNOTTING THE REINS

When performing exercises on the lunge, it is best to knot the reins so they do not become a safety issue.

Hold the reins near the buckle, both reins together.

Make a circle with both reins.

Slip the buckle under and pull the buckle through the circle.

Keep the reins slightly loose on the bit—if there is too much tension on the bit, your horse will be uncomfortable.

If the need arises, you can reach and grab the knot and once again have control of the rein.

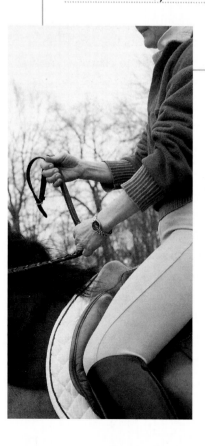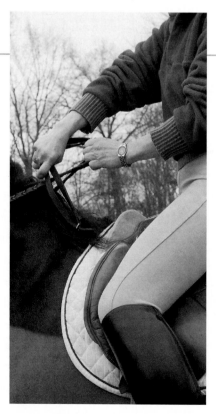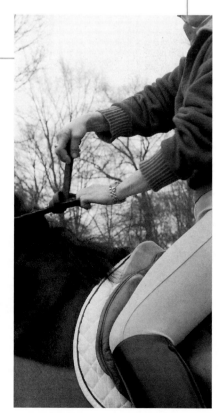

In order to allow the pelvis to have maximum freedom to follow your horse's movement, the thigh (femur) must be rotated inward. Before starting your ride, stand up in your stirrups and straighten your legs, so that your hips are above the pommel of the saddle. Gently inwardly rotate your thighs, one leg at a time, so that you are knock-kneed and pigeon-toed. Release down through your heels, and stretch your hips forward. Slowly slide down, bending at the hips and knees, and lower yourself into the saddle while keeping your thighs inwardly rotated. This will allow you to have a deep open seat, which means clearer communication for your horse.

EXERCISES AT THE WALK

CENTERING BREATHS

Calms, focuses and allows your horse move freely, prepares you and your horse for your ride.

Sit in the saddle and use the complete breath to center yourself.

Inhale into the upper ribs (clavicle), rib cage and then your abdomen.

Exhale from your abdomen.

Repeat 2-6 breaths.

SIDE STRETCH

Opens up the side of the body, expands the rib cage.

In a full seat, inhale and bring your right arm up alongside your ear.

Exhale as you slide your left hand down your hip and upper leg, stretching slightly to the right, opening up the space between your left shoulder and hip.

Keep your pelvis even, with weight on both seat bones.

Repeat to the other side.

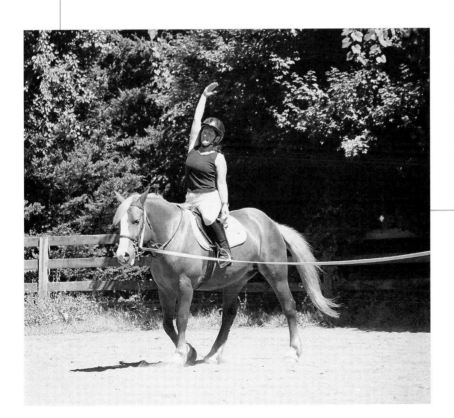

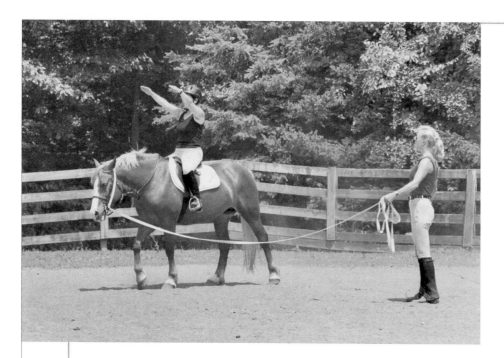

ARM CIRCLES

Opens the shoulders, relaxes the body and puts your full weight in your seat, while allowing your seat to move.

In a full seat, inhale and reach your arms out and forward (palms down), and then up in a backwards motion, feeling full movement through the shoulder.

Exhale and complete the arm circle. Perform the movements slowly and rhythmically.

Repeat 2-6 times.

Once you have some experience, you can use the complete breath while performing this exercise.

SEATED TWIST

Opens the front and sides of the body, relaxes the lower back. By turning your hands palm up, you open up your shoulder and chest.

In a full seat, inhale and bring your arms out to the sides, palms up. Feel the difference with palms up and the chest open, with the shoulder blades being able to slide down your back.

Exhale as you turn from your center slowly to right.

Inhale and return to center.

Exhale and turn slowly to the left.

Keep weight even in the seat bones—the twist is at the waist.

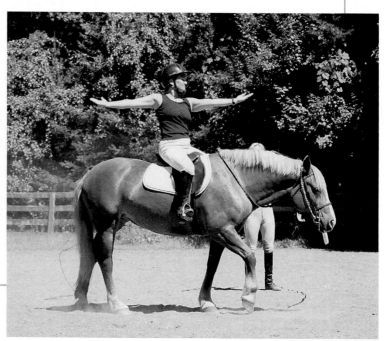

HALF CAMEL VARIATION
(A barn favorite, a delicious stretch)

Opens up the side of the body, stretching the obliques, and brings length into the side by stretching the shoulder away from the hip. The hand on the horse's croup should be moving into the arm and moving the shoulder girdle.

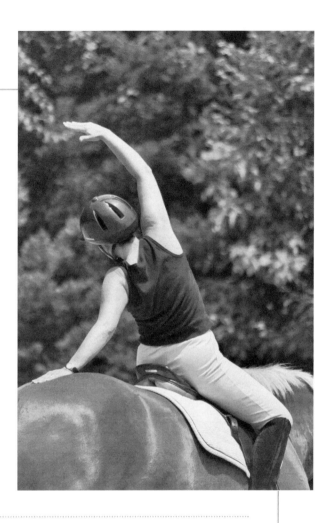

In a full seat, inhale and raise your arms out to the side, palms up.

Exhale and twist to the left and place your left hand palm down on your horse's croup, letting your elbow have a slight bend so that the movement of the horse moves your shoulder girdle.

Inhale and raise your right arm up and over your head, lifting your rib cage away from your hips. Feel how the thigh lengthens down and out from the hip; keep contact with your lower legs.

Turn your head in the direction of the twist and use deep breathing; with each inhale reach a little farther through the stretch.

Repeat to the other side.

BIRD BREATHS

Opens the shoulders, relaxes the back, and allows your horse to move freely.

In a full seat, inhale and raise your arms up and out to the sides, palms up, stretching and touching the fingers over the head.

Exhale and lower arms (feel the shoulder blade slide back down towards the spine), palms facing down.

Repeat 2-6 times.

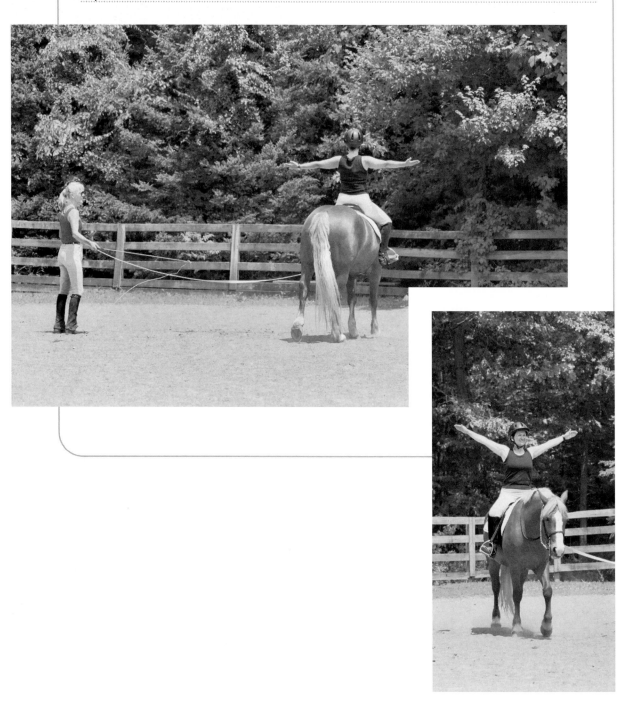

PUPPET/BOAT

Allows you to strengthen and bring awareness to your abdominal muscles while keeping your seat (balancing the bowl of your pelvis).

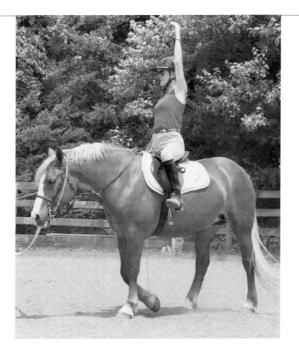
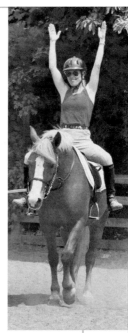

In a full seat, drop your stirrups, and let your legs hang freely.

Inhale and raise your left arm and leg (knee bent, lifting the thigh), keeping your back straight and your weight in your seat bones.

Exhale and lower your arm and leg.

Repeat to the other side.

Alternate 2-4 times each side.

Now inhale and raise both arms up and over your head as you raise both legs up, tightening your core (abdomen) to support your lower back. Pay attention to your hips and do not tighten through the hips, but let them move with the horse.

Exhale and lower arms and legs.

As you get stronger, stay for 2-6 breaths.

HALF SEAT

Brings awareness to the lower leg, and allows the arms to relax while opening the chest and shoulders.

In a full seat, inhale and bring your hands to your lower back, palms facing out.

Exhale and, using your lower leg, assume half-seat position, bringing hips up and forward.

Hold for several strides.

Move in and out of the posture gently.

Repeat 2-6 times.

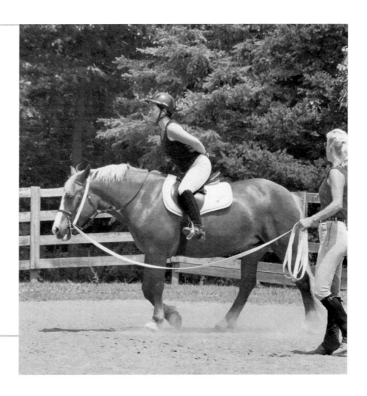

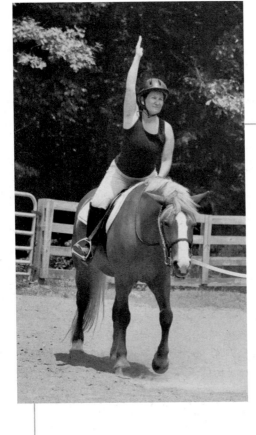

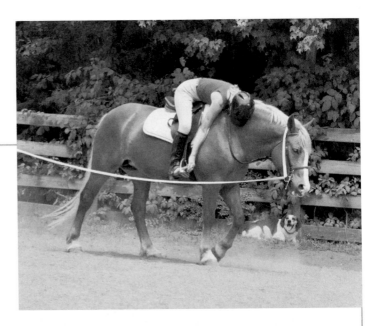

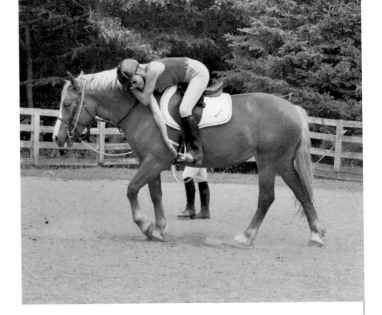

HALF-SEAT STRETCHES

Allows you to keep your weight in your heels while stretching the shoulders and upper back and pelvis.

Place your left hand on your horse's neck.

Inhale and bring your right arm up and forward (palm facing left), extending the upper back.

Exhale and bring your hand down to touch your toe, folding at the hips. Keep your lower back straight, with your hips over the middle of the saddle and your ankles under your hips. Stay for several breaths.

Inhale and raise your right arm up and forward again.

Exhale and thread your right arm under your left arm and towards your left toe, keeping your back flat and twisting the spine from the shoulders to the hips. Stay for several breaths.

Inhale and return to center.

Repeat to the other side.

EXERCISES AT THE TROT

CENTERING BREATHS

Calms, focuses and allows your horse move freely, prepares you and your horse for your ride.

Sit in the saddle and use the complete breath to center yourself.

Inhale into the upper ribs (clavicle), rib cage and then your abdomen.

Exhale from your abdomen.

Repeat 2-6 breaths.

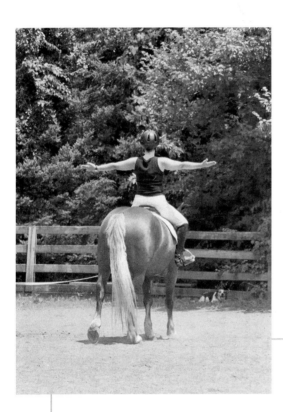
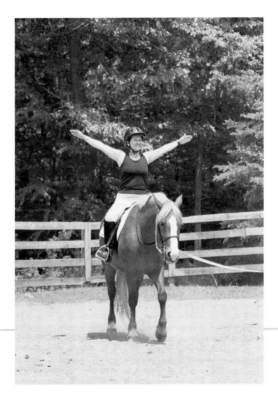

BIRD BREATHS

Opens the shoulders, relaxes the back, and allows your horse to move freely.

In a full seat, inhale and raise your arms up and out to the sides, palms up, stretching and touching the fingers over the head.

Exhale and lower arms, palms facing down.

Repeat 2-6 times.

SEATED TWIST

Opens the front and sides of the body, relaxes the lower back. By turning your hands palm up, you open up your shoulder and chest.

In a full seat, inhale and bring your arms out to the sides, palms up. Feel the difference with palms up and the chest open, with the shoulder blades being able to slide down your back.

Exhale as you turn from your center slowly to right.

Inhale to center.

Exhale and turn slowly to the left.

Keep weight even in the seat bones—the twist is at the waist.

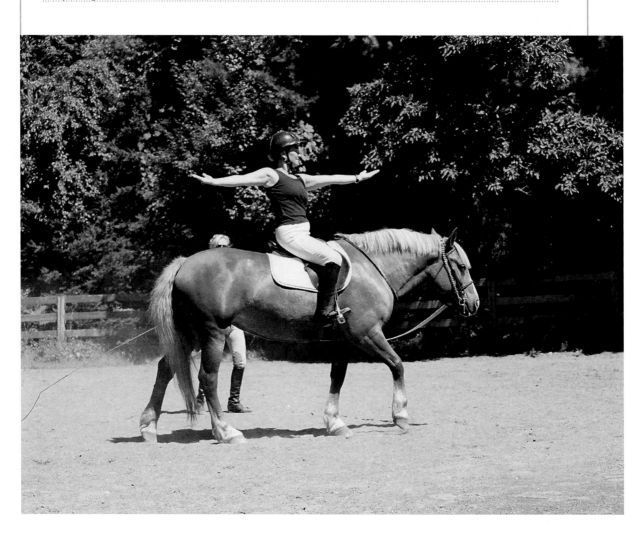

PUPPET/BOAT

Allows you to strengthen and bring awareness to your abdominal muscles while keeping your seat (balancing the bowl of your pelvis).

In a full seat, drop your stirrups, and let your legs hang freely.

Inhale and raise your right arm and leg (knee bent, lifting the thigh), keeping your back straight and your weight in your seat bones.

Exhale and lower your arm and leg.

Repeat to the other side.

Alternate 2-4 times each side.

Inhale and raise both arms up and over your head as you raise both legs up, tightening your core (abdomen) to support your lower back. Pay attention to your hips and do not tighten through the hips, but let them move with the horse.

Stay up for a few strides, and then exhale and lower arms and legs.

As you get stronger, stay for 2-6 breaths.

When raising both arms and legs at the trot, it is acceptable to hold on to the pommel with the outside hand for stability if needed. Make sure to practice each part of this exercise in both directions.

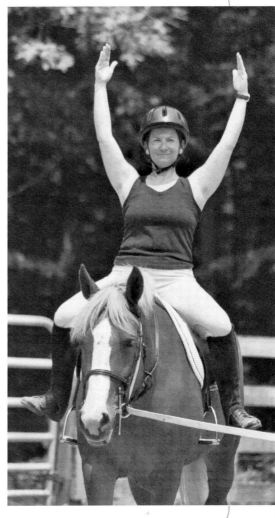

HALF SEAT

Brings awareness to the lower leg, and allows the arms to relax while opening the chest and shoulders.

In a full seat, inhale and bring your hands to your lower back, palms facing out.

Exhale and, using your lower leg, assume half-seat position, bringing hips up and forward. Hold for several strides.

Move in and out of the posture gently.

Repeat 2-6 times.

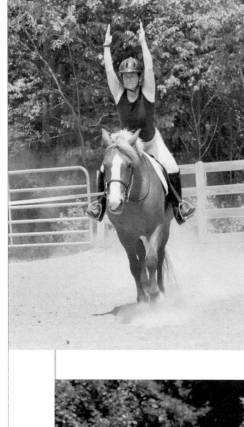

HALF-SEAT SEQUENCED FLOW

The flowing movement allows for relaxation and breath awareness while opening the shoulders, stabilizing the lower leg and strengthening the back.

In a half seat, inhale and bring arms out and up over head, palms facing.

Exhale and bring arms out to the side, palms up.

Inhale and bring arms up over head.

Exhale and bring arms out to the side.

Inhale and bring arms in front, palms facing.

Exhale and sweep arms out behind, palms facing out, opening the chest and sternum (sliding the shoulder blades towards each other).

Inhale and bring arms up over head, palms facing.

Exhale and fold forward, keeping your back flat (or you will lock your hips); you can rest your arms on the horse's shoulder, bending your elbows.

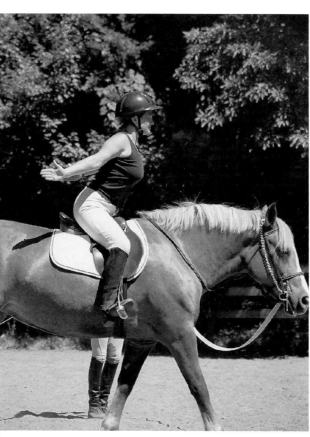

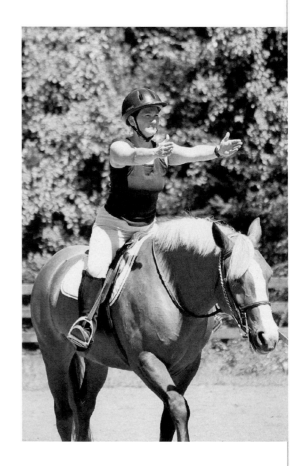

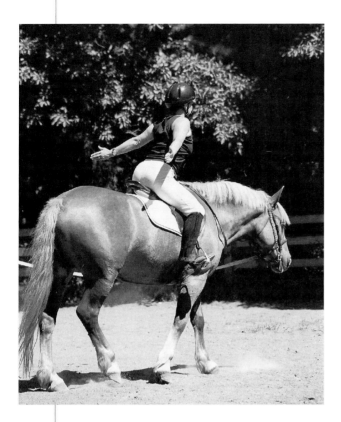

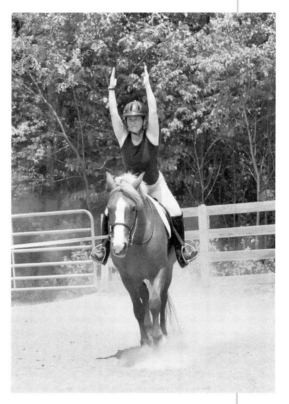

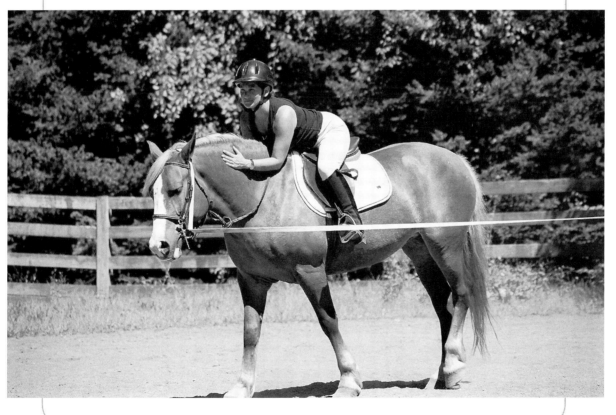

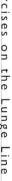

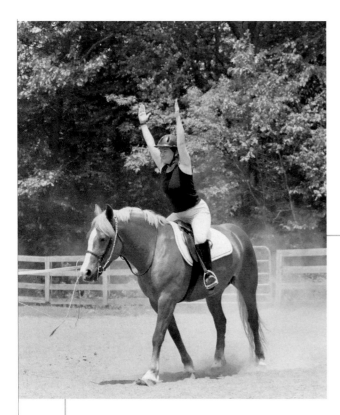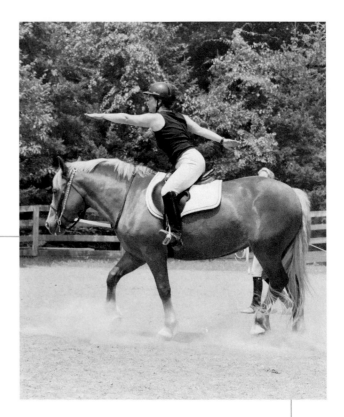

WARRIOR SERIES

Pairs breath with movement, relaxes the back and opens the sides and front of the body, brings awareness to your center and maintains balance and strength. Warriors are confident and brave—breathe into your confidence.

In a half seat, inhale and raise arms out and up over head, palms facing.

Exhale and bring your left arm in front and right arm behind you, twisting at the trunk, palms down.

Inhale and bring arms over up over head, palms facing.

Exhale and bring your right arm in front and left arm behind you, twisting at the trunk, palms down.

Repeat 2-6 times each side.

LOWER LEG AWARENESS

Strengthens the legs while bringing awareness of the importance of the lower leg for stability and balance.

Switch positions every 2-3 beats between full seat, half seat and posting.

Vary the sequence in order to focus on the importance of the lower leg when transitioning.

Keep your hands on your hips or lower back throughout the sequence.

LOWER LEG STRENGTHENER

Brings awareness to the lower leg and strengthens the legs.

Post and stay up for 2 beats.

Sit and stay for 2 beats.

Repeat.

HORSE AWARENESS

Brings awareness to the horse's movement and brings awareness to the horse's power center, the hind end.

Call off the strike of the horse's inside hind leg three consecutive times.

ENDING THE LUNGE EXPERIENCE

These exercises are performed at the halt, with someone holding the horse towards the head. They offer you a chance to challenge your balance skills.

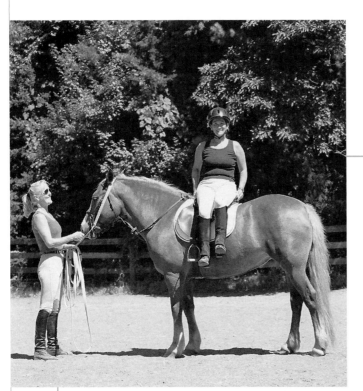

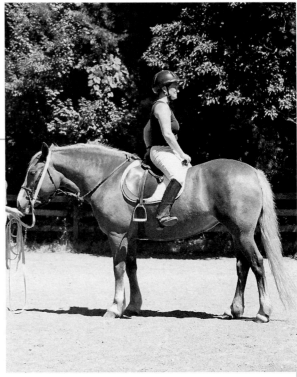

AROUND THE WORLD

Lift your right leg over the pommel to the left side, and then move from side-sitting to reverse by lifting the left leg over the cantle. Bring the right leg over the cantle and then the left leg over the pommel. Repeat in the other direction (clockwise).

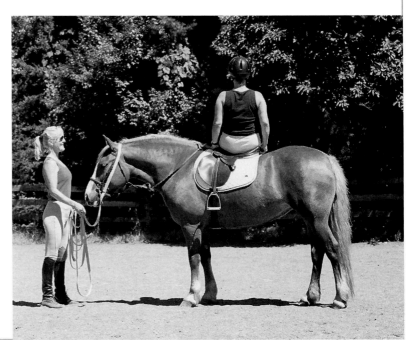

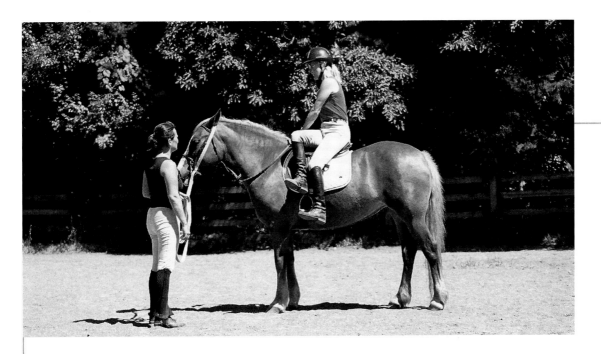

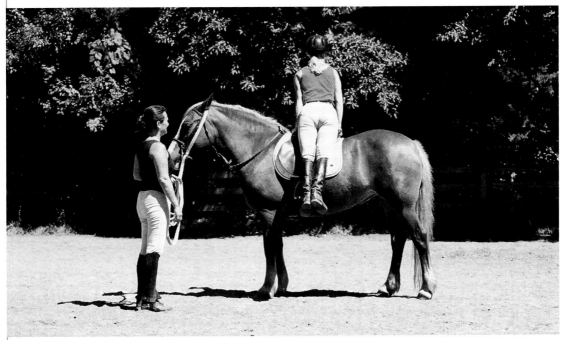

THREAD THE NEEDLE

Lift your right leg over the pommel so that you are side-sitting.

Rotate your trunk to the right and place your left hand on the pommel and right hand on the cantle.

Lift yourself up on the saddle and turn your body towards the horse.

Lift your body upwards and swing your right leg over the cantle to return to a sitting position.

Repeat in the other direction.

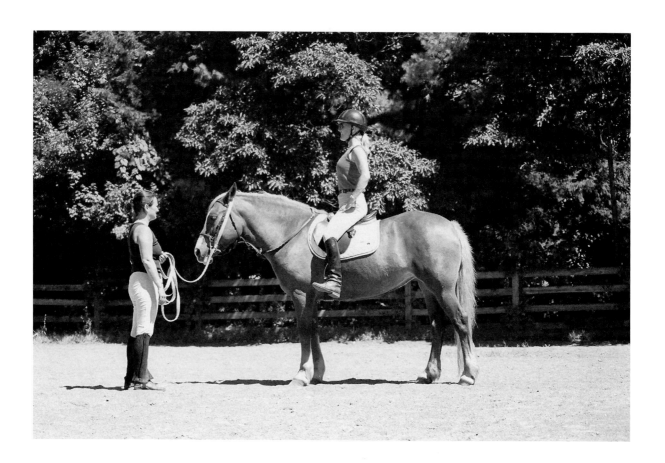

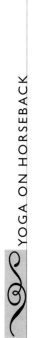

Chapter 6

Mounted Exercises

For the mounted exercises, you must be an independent enough rider to control your horse on your own, that is, without the lunge line. Your horse must be sensible and able to handle different situations, such as the different movements and release of contact from the bit. Not all horses are suited for yoga and riding. Please be vigilant when choosing the horse you are going to ride when performing these exercises. You should have experienced these exercises on the lunge prior to attempting them on your own.

Keep in mind what you have learned in the un-mounted and lunge line exercises. When performing exercises that involve both hands and require that you drop the reins, make sure the reins are knotted (see Chapter 5) so they do not fall over your horse's head and become a safety issue.

EXERCISES AT THE WALK

CENTERING BREATHS

Calms, focuses and allows your horse move freely, prepares you and your horse for your ride.

Sit in the saddle and use the complete breath to center yourself.

Inhale into the upper ribs (clavicle), rib cage and then your abdomen.

Exhale from your abdomen.

Repeat 2-6 breaths.

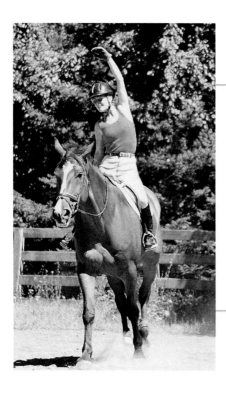

SIDE STRETCH

Opens up the side of the body, expands the rib cage.

In a full seat, inhale and bring your left arm up alongside your ear, holding the reins with your right hand.

Exhale as you stretch slightly to the right, opening up the space between your left shoulder and hip.

Keep your pelvis even with weight on both seat bones.

Repeat to the other side.

ARM CIRCLES

Opens the shoulders, relaxes the body and puts your full weight in your seat, while allowing your seat to move.

In a full seat, hold the reins with one hand and inhale and reach the other arm out and forward (palm down) and then up in a backwards motion, feeling full movement through the shoulder.

Exhale and complete the arm circle. Perform the movements slowly and rhythmically.

Repeat to the other side.

Knot and drop the reins, and circle both arms up and out, keeping your weight even on the seat bones.

Once you have some experience, you can use the complete breath while performing this exercise.

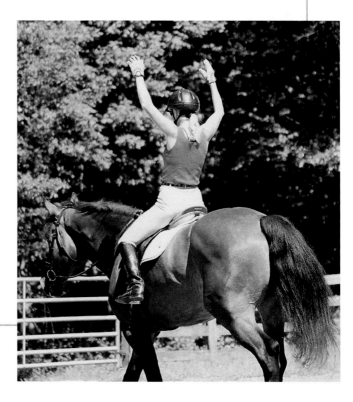

HALF CAMEL VARIATION

Opens up the side of the body, stretching the obliques, and brings length into the side by stretching the shoulder away from the hip. The hand on the horse's croup should be moving into the arm and moving the shoulder girdle.

Begin in a full seat, with reins knotted and dropped.

Inhale and raise your arms out to the side, palms up.

Exhale and twist to the right and place your right hand palm down on your horse's croup, letting your elbow have a slight bend so that the movement of the horse moves your shoulder girdle.

Inhale and raise your left arm up and over your head, lifting your rib cage away from your hips. Feel how the thigh lengthens down and out from the hip; keep contact with your lower legs.

Turn your head in the direction of the twist and use deep breathing; with each inhale reach a little farther through the stretch.

Repeat to the other side.

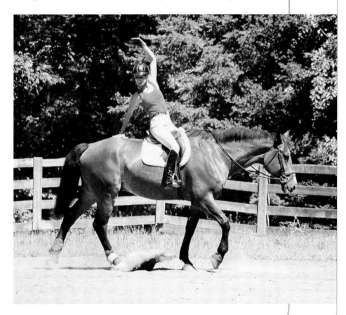

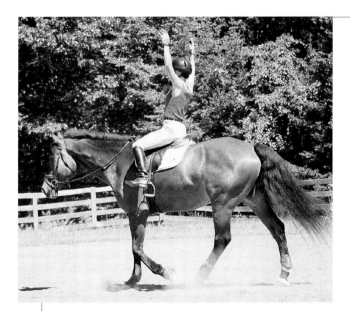

PUPPET/BOAT

Allows you to strengthen and bring awareness to your abdominal muscles while keeping your seat (balancing the bowl of your pelvis).

In a full seat, drop your stirrups, and let your legs hang freely.

Holding the reins in your left hand, inhale and raise your right arm and leg (knee bent, lifting the thigh), keeping your back straight and your weight in your seat bones.

Exhale and lower your arm and leg.

Repeat to the other side.

Alternate 2-4 times each side.

Knot and drop reins.

Inhale and raise both arms up and over your head as you raise both legs up, tightening your core (abdomen) to support your lower back. Pay attention to your hips and do not tighten through the hips, but let them move with the horse.

Exhale and lower arms and legs.

As you get stronger, stay for 2-6 breaths.

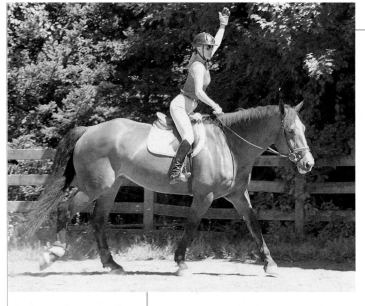

HALF-SEAT STRETCHES

Allows you to keep your weight in your heels while stretching the shoulders and upper back and pelvis.

Hold the reins in your right hand and place it on your horse's neck.

Inhale and bring your left arm up and forward (palm facing right), extending the upper back.

Exhale and bring your hand down to touch your toe, folding at the hips. Keep your lower back straight, with your hips over the middle of the saddle and your ankles under your hips. Stay for several breaths.

Inhale and raise your left arm up and forward again.

Exhale and thread your left arm under your right arm and towards your right toe, keeping your back flat and twisting the spine from the shoulders to the hips. Stay for several breaths.

Inhale and return to center.

Repeat to the other side.

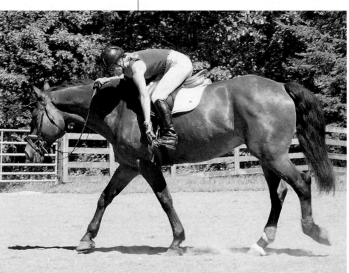

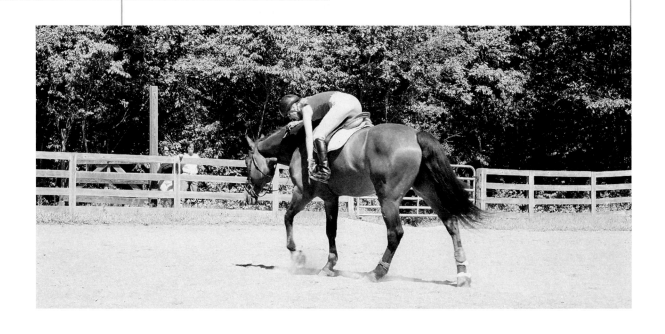

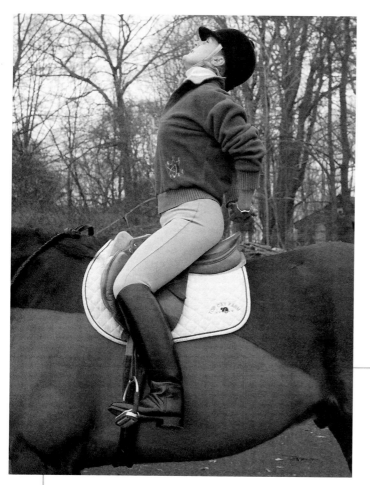

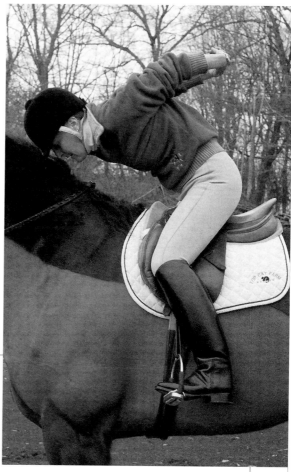

YOGA MUDRA

Opens up the shoulders and relaxes the neck.

Inhale and raise your arms out and up to the side.

Exhale and reach both arms behind you, clasping your hands together.

Inhale and then exhale and bring the shoulders down and back, slightly tip your chin so you are looking upwards.

Inhale and then exhale and bend forward at the hips, slightly rounding your back, and bring your clasped hands up behind your back.

Stay for several breaths.

Inhale as you rise up.

Exhale and release your hands.

Repeat 2-4 times.

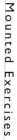

EXERCISES AT THE TROT

CENTERING BREATHS

Calms, focuses and allows your horse move freely, prepares you and your horse for your ride.

Sit in the saddle and use the complete breath to center yourself.

Inhale into the upper ribs (clavicle), rib cage and then your abdomen.

Exhale from your abdomen.

Repeat 2-6 breaths.

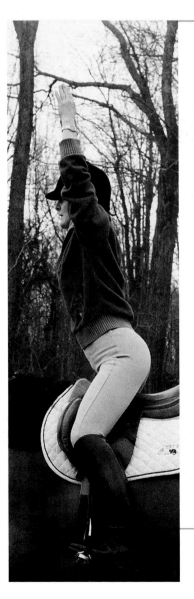

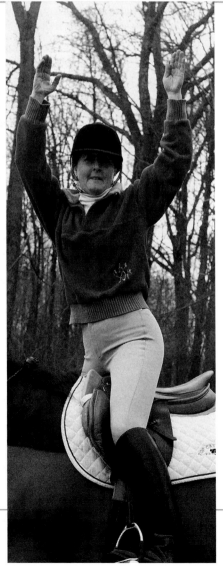

POSTING TWISTS

Helps your balance and brings awareness to your thighs.

Knot and drop reins.

While posting at the trot, inhale and lift your arms out to the side and up over head, hands facing each other.

On the rise of the trot, as you move your body up and forward, twist gently to one side from the waist.

Lower to the post.

On the next rise, twist gently to the other side. Keep the shoulders as soft and relaxed as possible.

WARRIOR I

Helps with leg awareness, evenness through the seat and legs, and feeling both sides of your body.

Knot and drop reins.

In a full seat, keep the horse centered between your legs as you inhale and raise your arms out to the side and up over head. Lift and open the rib cage.

Exhale and bring arms down.

Repeat 2-6 times, and then stay for several breaths.

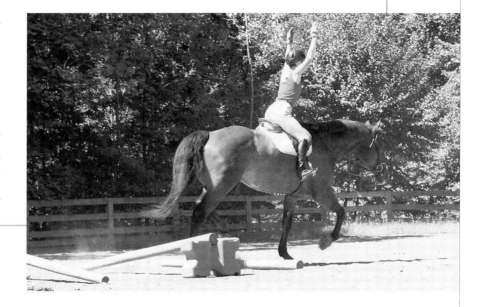

TROTTING POLES IN HALF SEAT

Brings awareness to your center and to the equal distribution of weight through your legs to navigate the horse evenly through the poles.

Exhale and move from full seat to half seat before getting to the poles.

Keep the horse centered between your legs as you go over the poles, letting your shock absorbers (hips, knees and ankles) work.

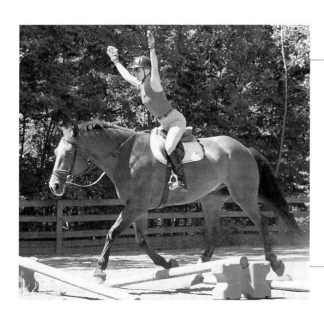

TROTTING POLES IN WARRIOR I

Knot and drop reins.

In a half seat, inhale and lift arms out to the side and up over head.

Breathe in and out in a natural pattern.

Gently lower arms once you are over the poles.

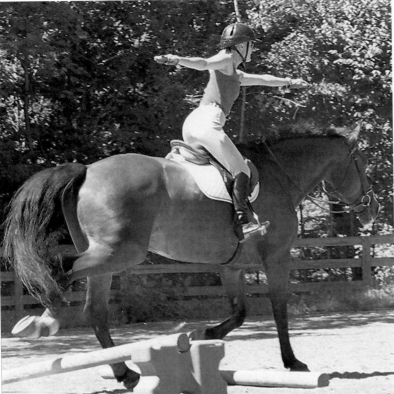

TROTTING POLES IN WARRIOR 2

With knotted reins, circle to go back over the poles.

Drop reins and rise into a half seat on the inhale and extend one arm in front and the other behind (Warrior 2) as you keep the horse between your legs over the poles.

Use full natural breaths over the poles.

Exhale, lower your arms and gently straighten once you're over the poles.

TROTTING POLES IN WARRIOR I VARIATION

In a half seat, with reins knotted and dropped, inhale and lift arms up and out to the sides with the palms facing up.

Use full, natural breaths over the poles.

Exhale and lower your arms, once over the poles.

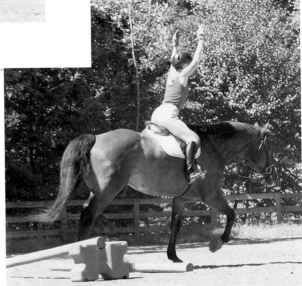

LOWER LEG AWARENESS

Strengthens the legs while bringing awareness of the importance of the lower leg for stability and balance.

Switch positions every 2-3 beats between full seat, half seat and posting.

Vary the sequence in order to focus on the importance of the lower leg when transitioning.

Keep your hands on your hips or lower back throughout the sequence.

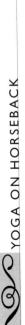

LOWER LEG STRENGTHENER

Brings awareness to the lower leg and strengthens the legs.

Post and stay up for 2 beats.

Sit and stay for 2 beats.

Repeat.

HORSE AWARENESS

Brings awareness to the horse's movement and brings awareness to the horse's power center, the hind end.

Call off the strike of the horse's inside hind leg three consecutive times.

EXERCISES AT THE CANTER

The Warrior postures (Warrior 1 and 2) can be performed by experienced riders at the canter. The rider must have a good seat and lower leg strength. The postures can be done down the long side of the ring and, for those looking for a greater challenge, while cantering over poles.

There are many variations to these exercises. Challenge yourself as you improve. Be aware and kind to your body and your horse. Feel a new openness and freedom through balance and breath. *Above all, have fun!!*

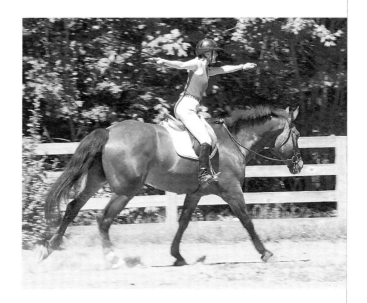

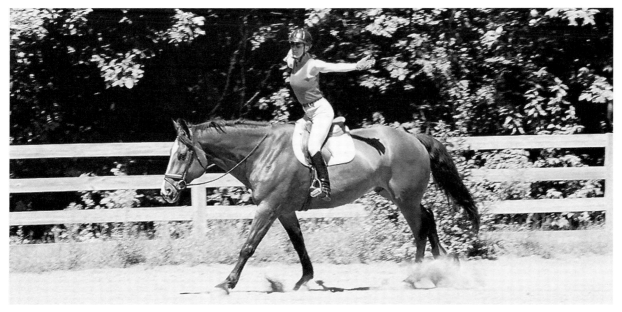

Glossary of Terms

Asana (*ah*-sah-nah)—a posture.

Ashtanga (*ash*-tahn-gah)—eight-limbed yoga; the way toward realization, based on Pantanjali's yoga sutras.

Hatha (*hah-tah*)—(ha = sun, tha = moon) the physical aspect of yoga designed to balance energy in the body.

Karma (*kahr*-mah)—action or the laws of action.

Mantra (*mahn*-trah)—a sacred word, thought or prayer; can be said aloud or silently.

Mudra (*muu*-drah)—a seal.

Nadi Sodhana (*nah*-de sho-*dah*-nah)—purification of the nadis (energy channels) through pranayama.

Patanjali (*pah-tahn*-jah-le)—the ancient sage who assembled the yoga sutras.

Prana (*prah*-nah)—breath, vital energy.

Raja (*rah*-jah)—mobility or activity; raja also means king.

Samadhi (*sah-mahd*-he)—bliss, state of bliss or union with the supreme; the final limb in the eight limbs of yoga.

Soft—describes muscles free from tension.

Sthirasukhamasanam (*shti*-rah-*suk*-hah-*mah*-sah-nam)—Yoga sutra II.46, translates as steady and comfortable posture.

Viniyoga (*vin*-e-yo-gah)—a style of yoga put forth and taught by TKV Desikachar; a type of yoga therapy working with each individual body.

Yoga Sutras (*yo*-gah *suu*-trahs)—an ancient text, put forth by the sage Pantanjali, that describes the way towards realization.

Bibliography/Suggested Reading

Benedik, L., and V. Wirth. *Yoga for Equestrians.* North Pomfret, VT: Trafalgar Square Publishing, 2000.

Desikachar, T. K. V. *The Heart of Yoga.* Rochester, VT: Inner Traditions International, 1999.

Farhi, Donna. *The Breathing Book.* New York: Henry Holt and Company, LLC, 1996.

Gillan, Lex. Yoga Teacher Training, July 2003, October 2004, April 2005.

Hafner, Stan. Yoga Teacher Training, July 2003, October 2004, April 2005.

Iyengar, B. K. S. *Light on Pranayama.* New York: Crossroad Publishing, 2002.

Iyengar, B. K. S. *Light on Yoga.* New York: Schocken Books, 1979.

Kraftsow, Gary. *Yoga for Wellness.* New York: Penguin Books, 1999.

Levine, Steven. *Guided Meditations, Explorations and Healings.* New York: Anchor Books, 1991.

Mohan, A. G. *Yoga for Body, Breath, and Mind.* Boston: Shambhala Publications, 2002.

Mohan, A. G., and I. Mohan. *Yoga Therapy.* Boston: Shambhala Publications, 2004.

Steiner, Betsy. *A Gymnastic Riding System Using Mind, Body and Spirit: Progressive Training for the Rider and Horse.* North Pomfret, VT: Trafalgar Square Publishing, 2003.

Sullivan, Johanna. Yoga Teacher Training, October 2004, April 2005.

Swift, Sally. *Centered Riding.* North Pomfret, VT: Trafalgar Square Publishing, 1985.

Wimala, Bhante Y. *Lessons of the Lotus.* New York: Bantam Books, 1997.

Wanless, Mary. *The Natural Rider.* North Pomfret, VT: Trafalgar Square Publishing, 1987.

ABOUT THE AUTHORS

NICOLE C. CUOMO has been a yoga practitioner for over twenty years. She was certified as a yoga instructor in July of 2003 and is registered with the Yoga Alliance and the International Association of Yoga Therapists. Since then she has been teaching yoga and meditation. She is also an occupational therapist and has a master's degree in psychology. Nicole has worked as a therapist for 15 years, focusing on pediatrics; she has expanded her practice using manual therapy techniques and yoga in working with adults and children with pain and orthopedic and neurological disorders. She is also a Professional Member of the American Hippotherapy Association. Nicole is the owner of Saldare Therapy and Yoga, LLC. She has been riding under the instruction of Marty Whittle for several years and has learned a great deal from Marty, her horses and her yoga practice.

MARTY WHITTLE is the owner, instructor and trainer at Top Cat Farm in Killingworth, Connecticut. She has been teaching for over twenty-seven years and is a member and state representative of ARIA (American Riding Instructors Association). She has ridden throughout her life in the United States and England, hunting and showing jumpers, hunters, dressage and eventing horses. Animals in general but specifically horses (and teaching) are her passion. She has been practicing yoga for several years and has found it invaluable to her riding, training and instruction. "I knew when I was very young this was what I wanted to do, and I am very blessed to have that dream fulfilled."

Additional Alpine Titles You Might Enjoy:

Horse Anatomy, A Coloring Atlas. Robert Kainer, DVM, and Thomas McCracken, MS.
An exceptional and unique way to learn horse anatomy, the physical systems of the horse, common ailments or conditions that may affect them, and why.

The Equine Arena Handbook: Developing a User-Friendly Facility. Robert Malmgren. If you want to set up a practice arena or revamp an old one that has poor drainage or footing, this book is a must!

Trail Training for Horse and Rider. Judith Daly. The complete book for recreational trail riders. Covers safety, trail hazards and obstacles, and how to condition, socialize and train a safe and dependable trail horse.

To the Nines: A practical guide to horse and rider turnout for dressage, eventing, and hunter jumper shows. Jennifer Chong. A valuable source for juniors and amateurs to learn the practical aspects of competion. Filled with useful tips and practical how-to for dress, clothing care, tack selection, care and cleaning, organizing the paperwork required, keeping your horse healthy on the road, and saving money. Chong is an HA rated pony club graduate who has won nationation awards in dressage and eventing.

Training for Trail Horse Classes: Train Your Horse to Compete Successfully. Laurie Truskauskas. Makes training for this popular class easy with step-by-step instructions.

Understanding Showmanship: Everything You Need to Know to Win in Showmanship Classes. Laurie Truskauskas. Conditioning, outfitting and training the horse and handler for all types of showmanship classes.

For Futher Information:

www.alpinepub.com

Alpine Publications
38262 Linman Road
Crawford, CO 81415

1-800-777-7257

Free catalog of horse and dog titles available upon request.